The Lyme Ease Survival Guidebook

Separating Facts From Fiction to Educate &
Empower Lyme patients

Jenn Hyla

ADVANCE PRAISE FOR THE LYME EASE SURVIVAL GUIDEBOOK

"Jenn Hyla's *The Lyme Ease Survival Guidebook* is a very well-written and no-nonsense approach to the all-too complicated topic of Lyme disease, co-infections, treatments, and controversies surrounding them all.

She comes from a pace of authority, being a Lyme patient herself, and though she leaves few stones unturned in the convoluted road to recovery, she paves it with easy-to-understand guidance that most neurologically impaired patients can understand.

She also doesn't shy away from the nuanced areas of mood, mindset and mental focus and how important those tools are to reaching complete recovery.

I would recommend this book to all newly-diagnosed Lyme patients."

- Gregg Kirk, CEO & Founder of Ticked Off Foundation & Lyme Recovery Clinic, Author of *The Gratitude Curve*

"As a Lyme Literate Psychotherapist, I understand how debilitating and isolating Lyme disease can be. To make matters worse, Lyme is hard to diagnose and difficult to treat.

Lyme is unlike any other disease, in which the patient MUST be knowledgeable and well researched to get proper care. There is too much conflicting information out there to leave your health care up to chance. This is why I am so impressed with Jenn Hyla's book, The Lyme Ease Survival Guidebook. This book will save you years of frustration, missteps, and needless suffering.

Jenn Hyla is a brilliant writer and researcher, and she understands the mysteries of Lyme disease firsthand. Jenn puts to good use her scientific background to figure out the shortest route to diagnosis, treatment and recovery of Lyme disease.

The Lyme Ease Survival Guidebook will help you to become an expert in the recovery of your own health!

- Brelan Armstrong, Lyme Literate L.C.S.W.

"*The Lyme Ease Survival Guidebook* provides a great overview of the issues and challenges surrounding Lyme disease.

It uncovers how to deal with those challenges in a holistic manner, along with providing a lot of great research to guide patients through the issues around chronic Lyme disease. A great read for anyone newly diagnosed or facing set-backs in their treatment."

- Lauren Lovejoy, President & Founder of Lyme Warrior

ISBN: 9798649616805

For the Lyme patient who refuses to give up on themself,
these words are all for you.

Never give up.

CONTENTS

          References   87

          Acknowledgments   103

          About the Author   104

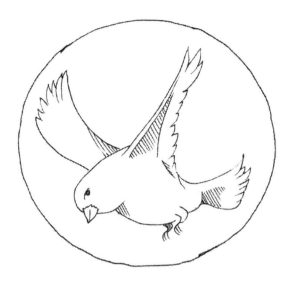

INTRODUCTION

Lying in bed unable to feel my arms and legs from a mysterious illness, I was almost fascinated by what was going on. If only it wasn't happening to me. I had been an active field biologist only weeks before. Now my body was completely shutting down. My doctors and I were stumped, as test after test came back negative.

As I was being referred from specialist to specialist, my health was declining rapidly. I began to lose cognitive abilities and developed vision problems. I lost my depth perception, and ability to drive. I can't tell you how many dishes I broke thinking the table was closer to me than it was. I developed a terrifying memory problem that my doctor called "intermittent amnesia." I was having daily panic attacks, and no one seemed to know what was happening.

Eventually, I went to see "the best gastroenterologist in the city." The guy had no bedside manner, and as I cried trying to explain the long list of symptoms I was going through, he bluntly suggested I ask my general doctor for a Lyme test. I remember leaving that appointment feeling like I had been blown off. I asked my doctor to do a Lyme test simply to rule it out. To my complete surprise, a few weeks later, I was told I had an unequivocally positive Lyme test. My first response was, "that can't be right, isn't Lyme an East Coast problem?"

"There is no arguing with this result," my doctor explained. The test had come back IgG, and IgM positive, meaning I had the acute and chronic markers for Lyme disease. I didn't know a thing about Lyme disease, but my doctor said that it could explain all the mysterious symptoms that I had been experiencing over the last 4 years.

Once I had the late-stage Lyme diagnosis, I imagined I'd be placed on some sort of healing conveyor belt. My doctors would surely know what to do. Now my only responsibility will be to rest and heal, I thought. Little did I know the diagnosis would only reveal one layer of a complex and controversial illness that would require complex treatment and years of healing.

HOW DO YOU GET LYME DISEASE?

Although, most commonly spread by tick bite studies are indicating that mosquitos, spiders, sand flies, and fleas may be capable of spreading Lyme disease.

In the book, *Healing Lyme*, Dr. Stephen Buhner, states,
"Although the number of spirochetes tend(s) to be lower in mosquitoes than in ticks, the spirochetes are established in them. Regular transmission through alternative routes such as mosquitoes, mites, and biting flies, although lower than that of ticks, does occur." [9]

It is likely that the majority of those who contract Lyme are infected by ticks in their first (larval) and second (nymph) stages of growth.

These ticks can be the size of the period at the end of this sentence, and their bite is completely painless.

The saliva of the tick contains numbing agents that allow them to stay attached up to several days unnoticed. Tick saliva also contains a cement-like material that hardens around the bite site. It is speculated that the unique compounds in tick saliva play a role in the transmission of Lyme disease, as studies done with needle inoculation in lab animals fail to produce the same results as tick bites do. [10]

Warmer winters have allowed for longer breeding seasons, and the world is seeing rapid spread and growth in both tick populations and Lyme disease.[11]

Once infected, a tick may pass pathogens to its 3,000 to 5,000 offspring, which can survive up to a year without a meal.

Ticks rarely carry *B. burgdorferi* alone, many Lyme patients discover they have several tick-borne illnesses referred to as co-infections. These co-infections can cause their own long list of symptoms as well.

The website tickencounter.org provides information to help identify the ticks and which illnesses are associated with each species of tick.[12]

B. burdorferi **transmission has also been recorded through blood transfusion, organ transplant, and congenitally passed from mother to fetus.**

Spirochetes can disseminate to any location in the body, and live spirochetes have been found in brain tissue, bone, saliva, tears, semen, and vaginal excretions. Sexual transmission is widely speculated in the Lyme community, but research is sparse, and animal studies have not proven sexual transmission possible.[13]

HOW LYME DISEASE WORKS

As the bacteria that cause Lyme disease, *B. burgdorferi*, enters the bloodstream in spirochete form, it begins to adapt quickly to the changes between multiple hosts and vectors.[14]

As the bacteria spreads throughout the bloodstream it begins to shed outer layer proteins which may confuse the body's immune system.[15] These proteins, known as blebs, can attach to healthy tissue which may also play a role in cases of persistent illness.

Dependent on many variables, such as the introduction of antibiotics, the spirochete form can metamorphose to completely lose its cell wall, by curling up into a cyst form.[16] This is a powerful defensive mechanism, as most antibiotics work by attacking the cell wall.[17]

Once in cyst form, it can also develop a biofilm to further protect itself from the immune system and antibiotics.[18] These biofilms become a microenvironment where many different bacteria and viruses can multiply.

No matter what stage or form the bacteria is in, the body's defenses are busy attacking the outer protein blebs, and bacteria, which disseminate throughout the body causing widespread inflammation.[19]

Lyme disease can be difficult to treat due to the bacteria's ability to change physical forms in response to its environment.[20] There is also some evidence to suggest that *B. burgdorferi* may alter its environment through gene expression. Recent studies conducted by naturopath and genetic counsellor, Dr. Bob Miller, indicate that chronically ill Lyme patients have higher levels of genetic variants.

In a 2016 research project titled "Higher Levels of Genetic Variants (SNPs) Found in those with Chronic Lyme Disease" he states:

"We examined 350 genes that are involved with mitochondrial function, methylation, neurotransmitter production, antioxidant production, and patterns that may result in excess production of oxidative stress, including superoxide, glutamate, ammonia and peroxynitrite. The data collected suggests unique genetic variations may be found in individuals with Chronic Lyme Disease."[21]

Although we began studying Lyme disease back in 1974, discoveries about this bacterial infection are being revealed every year.

Much more research is needed to determine how this complex illness truly works, and how to treat it.

HOW LYME TESTING WORKS

Tick Testing

First things first, if you are bitten by a tick, make sure to remove it properly. To do so, start by pulling it directly out by the mouthparts with a tick key or sharp tweezers. Never twist or put anything on a feeding tick. Never handle a tick with bare hands, as they are covered in pathogens. Always bag and save the tick for testing.

Tick testing is much more accurate than human testing and can yield pathogen results within days. Human testing is reliant on antibodies that may not show up for several weeks.

The website tickencounter.org is a great resource to find tick testing options in your area, and help you identify the tick.

Standard Blood Testing

The standard blood testing for Lyme disease is known as the two-tiered Western-blot test. First, a blood sample is tested using the EIA (Enzyme immunosorbent) / ELISA (Enzyme-Linked Immunosorbent Assay) method. This simple blood test is used for many different illnesses and is reliant on antibodies found in the blood sample.

The bacteria or virus (antigen) being tested for, in this case, *B. burgdorferi* is added to the petri dish. If antibodies are present in the blood they will bind to the antigen and produce a positive result. A positive ELISA test requires the sample to be further tested using the Western-Blot method. This looks for antibody reactivity to specific proteins found on *B. burgdorferi*.

The CDC previously required all 5 antibody bands to be present to determine positive results.[22]

Recently, both the FDA and CDC cleared a new ELISA test designed to detect *B. burgdorferi* known as the ZEUS EIA (enzyme immunoassay). This new test will take the place of the western-blot test as the second tier for Lyme testing.

"On July 29, 2019, [the] FDA approved several Lyme disease serologic assays with new indications for use based on a modified two-test methodology. The modified methodology uses a second EIA in place of a western immunoblot assay."
-CDC.gov[23]

Due to the stealthy nature of Borrelia, these antibodies are not always produced in the body, especially during the early stages, when treatment is critical.

The EIA/ ELISA blood test will turn up with false negatives 35% to 50% of the time.[24]

Many Lyme specialists will skip the ELISA and go right to Western blot or PCR testing which looks for specific proteins present in *B. burgdorferi*, rather than relying on antibody response.

There is another *big* problem with the standard blood test, once you have a positive antibody response for Lyme disease the body will continue making those antibodies for years.

The EIA testing method cannot be used to monitor the body's

response to treatments or determine if the bacteria has been eradicated.[25]

PCR Testing

Another option for Lyme testing is known as a PCR (Polymerase Chain Reaction) test. It is done through blood or urinalysis using a method known as amplification.

This method can detect small amounts of the bacteria or viruses' DNA within a sample.[26]

It can also detect several different strains of bacteria in one sample.[27] Unfortunately, this test is not currently accepted by the CDC for Lyme disease so most insurance companies will not cover it, and many doctors will not rely on the results to treat the disease.,

Ticks can also harbor many different types of bacteria, viruses, and parasites.

Each tick-borne infection comes with its own list of symptoms, some of them indistinguishable from Lyme disease making it difficult to recognize and diagnose. If Lyme treatments are not providing relief, you may be dealing with another tick-borne infection.[28]

EIA blood testing for co-infections is available, but similar to Lyme disease testing can be highly inaccurate. PCR testing through urinalysis offered by DNA Connexions labs can test for 11 different tick-borne microbes including:

- *Anaplasmosis phagocytophilium*
- *Borrelia burgdorferi*
- *Babesia divergens*
- *Bartonella bacilliformis*
- *Ehrlichiosis*

- *Borrelia recurrentis*
- *Borrelia miyamotoi*
- *Babesia duncani*
- *Bartonella henselae*
- *Babesia microti*
- *Bartonella quintana*

Clinical Diagnosis

Due to the wide variety of symptoms that manifest and the high incidence of false-negative testing, Lyme patients are often misdiagnosed multiple times.

The average Lyme patient reports two to five years before being properly diagnosed.[29]

Specialists known as "Lyme Literate Physicians" often clinically diagnose Lyme disease based on symptoms rather than relying on inaccurate diagnostic testing.

If you suspect your symptoms could be caused by Lyme disease, Dr. Richard Horowitz has created a symptom questionnaire to help you determine if you should start the search for a Lyme Literate Physician.

This is also a great tool to help you monitor your symptoms throughout treatment. It's available free on his website here: http://www.cangetbetter.com/symptom-list

HOW TO PROTECT YOURSELF FROM LYME

Lyme disease is the fastest spreading vector-borne disease in the world! Here are a few simple steps to help protect yourself.

Wear Repellent

Treating clothing and shoes with permethrin repels and kills ticks, mosquitos, and other pathogen spreading insects on contact. Permethrin is the synthetic version of pyrethrum, a natural insecticide derived from the chrysanthemum flower. It is considered non-toxic and authorized for use on clothing, outdoor gear, and dogs with the U.S. EPA.

> *Keep in mind that it is highly toxic to bees and other beneficial insects, fish, tadpoles, and cats. It is designed to last up to 6 weeks or 6 washes.*

I treat my clothing every 6 weeks with Permethrin and apply a topical insect repellent daily.

I like to use all-natural repellent made with essential oils and witch hazel. Here is my all-natural bug repellent recipe:

> In a 4 oz spray bottle, I combine 10 drops each - peppermint, lemongrass, cedarwood, eucalyptus, and tea tree essential

oils then fill with witch hazel. Shake well before each spray, and apply to exposed skin and clothing.

This recipe is not recommended for pets or children under 10.

Tick Check

Keep a lint roller in your car, and by the front door. Use the roller along your outer clothing before entering your home or car to remove any ticks. Put exposed clothing in the dryer on high for 7 minutes before washing, as ticks have been shown to survive within the threads of clothing through the washer and dryer up to 70 minutes.

Perform a proper tick check daily and after any outdoor activities.

This can be done by removing all of your clothing, using a mirror or a friend, in a well-lit area to thoroughly look at your entire body. Paying special attention to the scalp, behind the ears, knees, toes, and groin. Remember that nymph ticks can be the size of poppy seeds. They can easily be mistaken for a freckle. After you've checked every inch of your body, take a warm shower. This should be done within two hours of being outside.

If you do find a tick, make sure to remove it properly.

To do so, start by pulling it directly out by the mouthparts with a tick key or sharp tweezers. Never twist or put anything on a feeding tick. Never handle a tick with bare hands, as they are covered in pathogens. Always bag and save any ticks you find for testing and report it to www.tickencounter.org.

Treat Your Yard

Over the last few years, the world is seeing a massive rise in tick populations. Treating your yard can keep your home protected in high-risk areas.

There are many different ways to do this, but however you choose to do it, you'll want to treat your yard every few weeks during active insect seasons.

Tick-tubes are an easy and cost-effective way to reduce tick populations on your property.

To create tick tubes you will need empty toilet paper rolls, lint from the dryer or cotton balls, and permethrin. Wearing gloves in a well-ventilated outdoor area, treat the lint or cotton balls as directed on the permethrin bottle, and allow to dry. Stuff the treated material into the empty toilet paper rolls. Place these tick tubes along the perimeter of your property every few weeks. Since permethrin is not harmful to mammals or birds, the material will be taken back to rodent and bird nests and effectively kill and repel ticks.

Be aware that permethrin is harmful to aquatic life and honey bees. Never spray near flowering plants, or open water, and ensure your tick tubes will not roll into waterways. Wet permethrin is also toxic to cats.

Cedarwood chips and cedarwood essential oil can also be a powerful deterrent to many insects, including ticks. Treat your grass and garden by adding essential oils to water in a spray bottle or hose attachment. You can also create a natural insect barrier with cedarwood chips placed around wooded areas and the entry to your home or playground.

Diatomaceous earth is made of ground silica and is deadly to many insects. It is harmless to animals and humans but should be used with caution as the airborne dust can damage the lungs. I like to sprinkle a line of it near doorways, windows, and gardens as a natural insecticide to protect my home.

Know the Early Signs of Lyme Disease

As I mentioned at the beginning of the book, Lyme disease is known as "The Great Imitator." It is not always easy to recognize the early symptoms of Lyme disease.

Less than 50% of Lyme patients report a bulls-eye rash or recall a tick bite.

Tick bites are often painless, and other insect bites are often overlooked, so being aware of the early signs can increase your chances of proper diagnosis.

Be on the lookout for any flu-like symptoms - including fever and swollen-glands, headache, and stiff neck. Unexplained joint pain, neuropathy, and facial nerve dysfunction - often mislabeled as Bell's palsy. Lyme patients also report general pain or discomfort sensation throughout the body.

It is quite common for these early symptoms to be dismissed as a common cold or flu. Lyme disease should be suspected if any or all of these symptoms occur after a bug bite.

Always protect yourself with repellent, frequent tick checks, and trust your instincts.

Keep a copy of Dr. Richard Horowitz's symptom questionnaire, mentioned in the clinical diagnosis section, and check-in with yourself often.

Seek medical care as soon as possible if you believe you've been exposed to Lyme disease.

WHY IS LYME TREATMENT CONTROVERSIAL?

There is a lot to be said about the controversies that surround Lyme disease. To be honest, it could fill an entire book! So, I'm only going to cover the bits that I believe will help you in your healing journey. There are resources at the end of the book which you can use to dive deeper into the controversies that surround Lyme disease if you so choose.

When caught early, before the bacteria spread throughout the body, a short course of antibiotics may be all that is needed to wipe out *B. burgdorferi*. However, due to the bacteria's stealthy nature and defensive mechanisms, once the bacteria have disseminated throughout the body, the standard treatment for Lyme disease fails for many patients.

Despite thousands of peer-reviewed studies, and the medical community reporting high treatment and testing failures, the CDC has maintained its stance that Lyme disease is both easy to diagnose and easy to treat.

The CDC sanctioned Lyme treatment protocols do not consider the length of infection, symptoms, co-infections, or complications.

The CDC protocols state that if a Lyme patient is still experiencing symptoms past the prescribed 1 day to 28 days of antibiotic treatment, these symptoms are now caused by Post-Treatment Lyme Disease Syndrome (PTLDS).[30]

The CDC and Infectious Disease Society of America (IDSA) have little to say about PTLDS. I could not find any information on the first cases of PTLDS or who came up with the term. There is no medical billing code for patients diagnosed with PTLDS, and there are no treatment recommendations by the CDC.

There are very few federally funded research projects being done on PTLDS, and the only treatment mentioned on the CDC website is time and symptom management at your doctor's discretion.

"Patients with PTLDS usually get better over time, but it can take many months to feel completely well. If you have been treated for Lyme disease and still feel unwell, see your healthcare provider to discuss additional options for managing your symptoms."
-CDC.gov[31]

If your doctor continues to treat you for Lyme disease outside of the CDC protocol they may be held liable for "unprofessional conduct" and can be sued by insurance companies.

Many Lyme treating physicians have gone bankrupt and even had their medical licenses suspended for treating outside of the CDC guidelines.[32]

With high treatment failure rates and harsh penalties for treating outside treatment protocols, you can imagine why many doctors might be reluctant to treat Lyme disease.[33] I had to call over 35 different infectious disease doctors before one would see me with my positive Western blot Lyme test in 2015.

Lyme advocacy groups, scientists, and many doctors disagree with the CDC's protocol and description of PTLDS, and the handling of Lyme disease.

A recent study on patients with chronic Lyme found measurable and widespread brain inflammation after failing antibiotic treatments, suggesting that PTLDS may be caused by persistent infection.[34]

The International Lyme and Associated Diseases Society (ILADS) has created a training program for doctors to become knowledgeable about the complications of Lyme disease, and they all agree that treatment should be dictated by how the patient feels.

"Many patients with early Lyme have been treated with short courses of antibiotics (< 20 days) and recovered. However, both in practice and in the scientific literature, it has been observed that a significant number of patients do not return to their pre-Lyme health with short courses of antibiotics. The ILADS guidelines working group reviewed the available research and developed recommendations based upon the best available evidence, clinical expertise, and patient-centred values."
-ILADS.org[35]

Find A Lyme Specialist

Due to the controversies surrounding treatment, finding a Lyme Literate physician early on is crucial to creating a treatment plan.

A Lyme Literate Medical Doctor (LLMD) is a licensed physician who has gone through a training course with ILADS. ILADS trained physicians follow patient-centered treatment protocols, and go through a 2 weeks training course, but that doesn't mean they have all the answers.

Just like all medical professionals, there are both good ones... and some not so good ones. Most LLMDs cannot bill insurance and charge large cash fees, so be sure to research your options and follow your gut instincts.

ILADS provides referrals on its website ILADS.org to help you find a Lyme Literate physician in your area. They will email you three randomly selected options within a selected radius of your zip code.
https://www.ilads.org/patient-care/provider-search/

Before you go through the ILADS referral process, which offers randomly selected doctors, I recommend searching for a local Lyme disease support group. Facebook groups are a fantastic resource to connect with other Lyme patients in your area and see which doctors they are seeing.

Remember, that as people heal they tend to stop showing up in these online spaces. Limit your time to crowdsourcing answers to your specific questions. It is easy to get swept away with everyone else's experiences.

Don't forget that each person is affected differently, so what works for one person may not work for others.

Full healing may require multiple doctors, so don't be afraid to move on if you're not feeling heard or seeing results. In my healing journey, I found each doctor could only get me so far before they seemed to run out of ideas.

Make sure to check in with yourself after each appointment, and ask:

- Did I feel heard and respected?
- Did I leave the appointment feeling confident and supported, or confused and dismissed?
- Were my top concerns addressed?

Intentional Emotional Support

On top of all the physical symptoms, living with Lyme disease can feel very isolating and depressing. As we get sick our needs and boundaries drastically change, and in many cases, our relationships struggle to change with them.

Before my illness, I had a tight-knit group of friends that I considered my "ride or dies." As I began treatment, I also began to lose lifelong friendships in a painful and surprisingly fast way.

Losing friends and relationships due to Lyme disease was unexpected, but happened in what seemed like rapid-fire succession. Pretty much everyone I speak to in the Lyme community has similar stories.

Chronic illness of any kind has a major impact on relationships of all sorts, and the question so many people raise is, why? Why are seemingly solid friendships so easily wiped away in the throes of chronic illness?

I have a few ideas as to why relationships fail while facing chronic illness or crisis:

1. With chronic illness, our needs and boundaries drastically and suddenly change. Most of us expect our relationships to seamlessly change along with them. I think I had expectations of people to show up for me in ways they never had to before. I expected them to do what I imagined I would do if the roles were reversed, but never had that conversation with them.

So, when they didn't show up for me in the ways I needed, I became resentful. And likewise, when I couldn't show up for them in the ways I always had, they became resentful.

2. People can be extremely uncomfortable and even repelled by vulnerability and need for support because they are terrified of their vulnerability. My friends didn't have the skill set to support me because they have never truly faced or embraced their own needs.

A New York Times article suggests the more vulnerable people feel, the harder it may be to connect...many times people can picture all too vividly the same thing happening to them or their children. They feel too much empathy rather than not enough.

Psychologist Dr. Jackson Rainer, Ph.D., ABPP describes this kind of distancing as "stiff-arming" — creating as much space as possible from the possibility of trauma. It's magical thinking in the service of denial: If bad things are happening to you and I stay away from you, then I'll be safe.

Such people often wind up offering what Dr. Rainer calls pseudo-care, asking vaguely if there's anything they can do but never following up.

It's important to have an honest heart-to-heart with your loved ones. Be as honest with them about your condition as you can so they don't have to guess what's happening – or worse – assume it's nothing.

Invite them to ask questions when they don't understand something. Oftentimes, people will remain silently confused because they are afraid to set you off by asking. Allow for genuine questions of understanding and curiosity.

Set expectations both ways. Like I said, needs and boundaries change quickly but most people aren't capable of understanding or keeping up with those changes.

Let your loved ones know what you can and can't do anymore and why.

Ask them for specific ways they can support you. This leaves them with options and allows the relationship to begin shifting from its previous patterns. Maybe you can't go out with them much anymore, but they can come to visit you. Maybe your finances won't allow for road trips or movie nights, but you can plan potluck dinner and movie nights at each other's houses.

Make sure you give people a chance to catch up to your new reality, and they will be more likely to seek understanding about what is happening to you.

No matter how you tackle the issue of changing relationships in your illness, it's important to remember to take nothing personally. I know, it is seemingly impossible in the moment of rejection.

But over time, it will help you a great deal to know that people's reactions to your illness are always more about them and their stuff than you and yours. Their rejection often comes from a place of unprocessed fear which can breed all kinds of ugly outcomes.

Practice self-care and practice it often. I'll be writing more on this in a few chapters! For now, remember that taking care of your emotional, physical and spiritual needs is paramount to feeling better and being able to cope with the inevitable slopes you will go through.

Keep in mind that the inflammation from this illness can dramatically affect our mood and emotions.

For some, Lyme can manifest in depression, anxiety, sharp mood swings, and other psychological symptoms.[36] Oftentimes our friends and family members don't have the skill set to support us.

It can be nearly impossible to think rationally in the midst of psychological symptoms, so do not take emotional support lightly. The biggest killer of Lyme patients is not from physical complications, but suicide.

Take charge, and ensure you have a good support system. Have a plan in place for times you are in crisis and write it down.

I have an anxiety attack checklist with steps to take, people to call, songs to play, essential oils to use, and a guided meditation recording.

Pay more attention to how you feel, and what you're putting

energy into. Spend more time with compassionate and inspiring people that feel good to be around. Distance yourself and let go of toxic relationships that feel draining and insincere. Seek out emotional support from your local Lyme community, churches, community centers, and loved ones often. Find an understanding therapist, coach, or mentor you can speak to regularly.

Don't waste energy trying to do everything on your own, if you need help start asking! But don't inhibit your healing by getting upset with people who do not have the skill set to support you.

Find Financial Support

During treatment, it's important to get enough rest, and many patients find it difficult or impossible to work. The financial burden of Lyme disease is a big source of stress for many, and just like all stress, it will inhibit healing.

If you don't have enough savings to take extended time off work, below are a few ideas to ease the burden while undergoing treatment.

Patient grants and medication assistance programs are available through non-profit organizations across the United States, and internationally.

The Global Lyme Alliance has a current list of organizations offering Lyme patient grants and assistance programs available on their website. https://globallymealliance.org/financial-assistance/

Fundraising sites are an easy way for your friends and family to help out! Work on condensing your story into a few compelling paragraphs and ask someone to proofread it for you. Have a little photoshoot selfie party. That's everything you need for an online fundraiser!

Make sure you read the fine print on processing fees and

select an online fundraiser through GoFundMe, YouCaring, or any of the other thousands of sites that are popping up these days.

Advertising your fundraiser takes energy and shameless self-promotion, so try to get a group of family and friends together to help you share on social media, and within your community.

If you will be out of work for a year in the United States, you can apply for Social Security Disability(SSDI), a social security program that pays monthly benefits to those who are unable to work.

You must be found medically eligible, and have met payment standards into the Social Security (FICA) tax system. The filing process is tedious and can take years. I recommend working with a lawyer to help you start the process.

If your SSDI case is denied or you are struggling financially while waiting on the filing process, you may apply separately for Supplemental Security Income (SSI).

SSI is a federal program that pays monthly to assist low income disabled, blind, and aged individuals to help meet basic living needs. You may apply while waiting on your disability case to process. Here is a website that can help you determine if you qualify for Social Security benefits. https://ssabest.benefits.gov/

There are many other federal, state, and local assistance programs also available. If you are struggling financially, be sure to search for your local low-income programs.

Online resources like the Buy Nothing Project, MeetUp, church organizations, and other giving groups can connect you with generous neighbors to help with meal prep, chores, rides, and other favors.

You may have to get creative to make ends meet.

With the internet, nearly any talent can be monetized these days. So, consider creating an online business from home while you're healing.

Websites like Redbubble.com, Society6.com, and Etsy.com can help you to sell arts and crafts. Rover.com, Care.com, or Pettsitter.com can help you find house sitting and pet sitting gigs easily. Fiver.com, Freelancer.com, Flexjobs.com offers a variety of flexible and online work

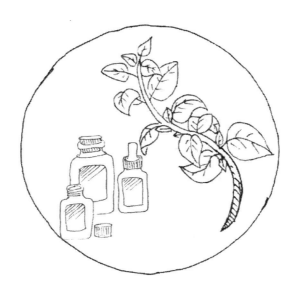

PART 2 ~ LYME TREATMENT OPTIONS

Lyme disease and co-infection treatments can get complicated. To avoid the hostile antibiotics and natural defenses of the immune system, the bacteria, *B. burgdorferi* deploys defensive maneuvers, shedding blebs, turning into cysts, hiding out in biofilm, and burrowing into blood cells, joints and tissues.[37]

The bacteria that do die-off from treatment release an onslaught of toxins into the bloodstream. These toxins may cause an overload to the system, and lead to a condition known as a Jarisch–Herxheimer reaction, more commonly referred to as a Herxheimer or Herx.

Herx reactions cause widespread inflammation and an increase in overall symptoms.

It can be very uncomfortable and debilitating for hours or days. In extremely rare cases, Herx reactions can cause a stroke or heart attack.[38] Most Lyme patients find supporting the detoxification system greatly reduces these reactions and eases symptoms throughout treatment. I'll be sharing my favorite detoxification support methods in a few pages.

Most ticks are carrying multiple pathogens along with the bacteria that causes Lyme disease. These other pathogens known as co-infections may be resistant to the antibiotics used to target *B. burgdorferi.*[39]

It's important to find a doctor familiar with the symptoms of all co-infections to help you address the multiple layers that come along with Lyme disease.

Since everyone is affected so differently by Lyme disease, I don't believe there is a prewritten treatment protocol that suits everyone. However, through my research, personal trials and experience working with other Lyme patients, I believe the most successful treatment plans accomplish the following:
- Reduce pathogens
- Address Biofilms

- Reduce inflammation
- Support detoxification
- Heal the gut
- Cultivate a healing mindset

I will go through what I've learned on each of these over the next few pages.

REDUCING PATHOGENS

There are many ways to combat the bacteria that cause Lyme and other tick-borne illnesses. Due to the variety of pathogens and individual responses to medications, I have included what I believe are the most common approaches.

This is not a treatment suggestion, nor a comprehensive list. Remember the information provided here is for educational purposes and meant to help you work with a qualified Lyme Literate Physician. Always research any new medications thoroughly.

Common Antibiotic Protocols

Infectious Disease Society of America (IDSA) protocol: 1 to 28 days of antibiotic protocol recommended by the IDSA and CDC. This protocol is considered by Lyme experts to have extremely low success rates, ranging from 52% to 84%.

Be aware that most infectious disease doctors follow the IDSA

naturally produced stem cells.

Recent studies are showing that prolonged fasting increases the flow of stem cells in the body.[48]

Clinical studies suggest that prolonged water fasting for 48 to 72 hours can have inexplicable healing benefits for the body.[49]

Although how it works is still largely a mystery, fasting is one of the oldest healing modalities on Earth. There are several clinics and doctors around the world, such as the True North Health Center, that offer medically monitored prolonged fasts.

ADDRESSING BIOFILM

When I first heard about biofilms I thought they were specific to Lyme bacteria, but I couldn't have been more wrong! They are in fact created by many different bacteria in many different environments.

They were first described in 1684 using simple microscopes by a Dutch scientist. His discovery proved for the first time that bacteria do not just flow freely through the bloodstream, it adheres to surfaces by creating these "surface-associated microbial cells."[50]

Further study wasn't done until 1973, when the electron microscope was invented, which provided higher magnification. With the new technology, studies were conducted on dental plaque, aquatic environments, and industrial water systems.

These studies showed that biofilm *were not only very tenacious but also highly resistant to disinfectants such as chlorine.*" Based on those studies the first theory of how biofilms function was created in 1978.[51]

Since then, we have discovered that each microbial biofilm is actually a community. Biofilms are not a single layer of surface deposits with one bacterial inhabitant. They are a microcolony of different bacterial cells, each one with unique structures.

Biofilms are a protective shield for the bacteria harbored inside. They are impenetrable by the immune system, and highly resistant to antibiotics.[52]

Only specialized compounds have been found to dissolve biofilms. *In vitro* testing has shown that a number of herbs, essential oils, and some antibiotics can be effective and are commonly referred to as "biofilm busters" in the Lyme community.

Small clinical studies on Lyme patients indicate that taking a "biofilm buster" can improve the effectiveness of antimicrobials or antibiotics.[53]

As always, I recommend working with your doctors to help you determine which "biofilm buster" to use and when. Ensure you're detoxing well because as you break up the biofilm, bacteria, fungi, and viruses that were inside can float free and overwhelm the body.

REDUCING INFLAMMATION

Inflammation is the body's natural process to flush an injured area with fresh blood and oxygen, as well as infection-fighting white blood cells. While short-term, acute inflammation is an important part of healing from traumatic injury to the cells or tissue, chronic inflammation is believed to lead to chronic disease.

The outermost layer of a human cell is called the plasma membrane. In a healthy cell, the plasma membrane protects it from its environment and selectively allows nutrients and waste to flow both in and out of the cell.

A sick cell has toxins, bacteria, viruses, and other pathogens sticking to the membrane blocking waste from leaving the cells. The energy-producing mitochondria, inside the cell, becomes inflamed, and cannot produce the energy and antioxidants the body needs. The cumulative waste and inflammation inside the cell can impact the DNA inside, and each replication or these sick cells are how chronic diseases of all kinds are believed to begin and progress.[54]

Simple changes in lifestyle and diet can reduce inflammation and ultimately improve the function of your cells.

Here is what I do to keep my inflammation in check.

1. Eat an anti-inflammatory diet. This is one of the most beneficial things a Lyme patient can do. Nutrition is medicine! Shifting the diet towards whole unprocessed foods will shift and strengthen your gut microbiome nourish your cells, and immune system.

Diet is so important that several Lyme specialists have gone on record to say they will not work with anyone unwilling to change their diet.

Foods rich in omega-3 fatty acids, and natural antioxidants, like whole fruits and vegetables can reduce inflammation and feed your cells what they need to heal. Refined sugar, starches, processed grains, and saturated fats have been shown to promote inflammation.[55]

Diet may also play an important role in our mental health. The book Gut and Psychology Syndrome uncovers the fascinating gut-brain connection and provides many healing recipes to help you make the switch to an anti-inflammatory healing diet.

2. Anti-inflammatory supplements. Along with eliminating inflammatory foods and improving nutrition, supplementing my diet made a huge difference in my cognitive function, pain and energy levels. Essential oils, herbs, and supplements can make a big difference for Lyme patients.

Here are a few of my favorite supplements:

- Fish-oil
- Boswellia / Frankincense
- Turmeric
- Copaiba

- Collagen
- Black seed oil
- Olive oil

3. Grounding. One of my favorite ways to reduce inflammation is by grounding, also known as earthing. Grounding is done by simply touching the earth with your bare skin. It may sound a little woo, but consider that every cell in our body has a positive and negative electrical charge.[56] The Earth and everything on it also has an electrical charge.[57]

Our rubber-soled shoes keep us insulated from the earth. Most of us go entire days and weeks without ever stepping foot on the earth un-insolated by shoes, concrete, and asphalt.

Studies done with thermal cameras have shown impressive reductions in inflammation. Study participants report drastic drops in stress and pain levels within just a few minutes of grounding.[58] Spending just 20 minutes a day in a space that lets you feel connected with nature can also reduce the stress hormone cortisol, which is strongly linked with inflammation.[59]

4. Cold water therapy. A simple yet powerful way to reduce inflammation, and manage pain is to simply turn your tap to cold in the shower. The science behind cold water therapy is astonishing. Just 1 to 2 minutes of cold water plunge or shower can flush the lymph system, constrict the circulatory system, burn fat, stimulate the immune system, and reduce inflammation.[60] Daily cold showers may also combat depression.[61]

After learning the benefits, I knew I had to give it a try! As someone who hated the cold, I didn't think I could keep it up, but to my surprise, I became hooked. Now, I've been taking cold showers for over two years. This practice lifts my fatigue, brain fog, and chronic pain, it has changed my life and I don't think I will ever stop!

If you decide to try it, read up on the benefits, it will help motivate you to get started. Once you're ready I recommend starting with a normal warm shower, then step away from the stream of water and turn to cold. Slowly exhale as you dip one body part into the cold water at a time. Making sure to control the breath and stay relaxed. Get out of the shower before you feel cold. Aim for 15 to 30 seconds of cold water at the end of your warm shower at first, and incrementally work your way to 1 minute or more slowly over time.

5. Time-restricted eating. What you eat is just as important as when you eat it. The body has its own internal clock, a 24-hour schedule known as the circadian rhythm that every single cell in our body runs on. Different processes occur, and hormones are released throughout the day to keep every system of the body running.

Scientists still have a lot to learn, but recent studies indicate that eating at times out of sync with the circadian rhythm, observed in shift workers, and jet lag, greatly disrupts the release of insulin and other digestive processes. This throws off the body clock which can lead to an increase in inflammation, problems sleeping, and a whole host of potential health problems.[62]

Following a circadian rhythm schedule is a great way to support your digestive system. Experts like Dr. Rhonda Patrick, of Found My Fitness, recommend a 16-hour window of fasting each day.[63]

This may sound like a challenge, but it can be accomplished fairly easily. A common method is to stop eating 4 hours before bed, sleep for 8 hours, and drink only water and black tea or coffee for 4 hours upon waking.

Of course, life may get in the way, so don't beat yourself up if you can't follow this schedule perfectly. The goal is to feed the body with nutritious foods when your digestive juices are highest and give yourself several hours to digest before bed.

6. Improve sleep. The body goes through many regenerative processes while we sleep. Studies show that adults need at least 7 hours of sleep for the body to fully flush toxins from the blood and brain.[64]

Studies in sleep-deprived mice indicate the detrimental effects on the immune system with measurable drops in immune-cell number and cytokine production.[65] The mice put through these experiments do not die of exhaustion, they actually die of infection.

One symptom most Lyme patients have in common is trouble sleeping. Whether they sleep for 16 hours or 2, they never feel fully rested. I always have my clients begin by getting intentional with their sleep.

Set yourself up for success with a relaxing evening routine, with limits on screen time during the last two hours before bed. This simple practice can help you get to sleep more easily. A daily evening routine can release the stress of the day and signal to the brain that it is time to rest. Studies show restorative yoga practices focused on relaxing and connecting with the breath can dramatically reduce the stress hormone cortisol.[66]

I know many people have grown accustomed to sleeping right next to their phones. It's often the last thing looked at each night, and the first thing looked at each morning. So, I want to talk a little more about the reasons time away from the screen can be beneficial.

First off, the blue light from the digital screens register as daylight to our primal brain, and it can signal our brain to stay awake. If you're tossing and turning, reaching for a smartphone could keep you awake for hours.[67]

Secondly, our subconscious mind is always absorbing information. Wearing blue-blocking glasses cannot block out the endless stream of content, and more importantly, stress, associated with social media or online games.[68]

Be intentional about the time you spend online. Use apps or timers to track the time you stare at the screen.

One last reason to stay unplugged each night is to reduce the exposure to EMF radiation and WiFi signals constantly emitted by smartphones. Many studies, explored in the 2017 article, Wi-Fi is an important threat to human health indicate oxidative stress, DNA damage, apoptosis, and endocrine changes possible from Wi-Fi and EMF exposure.[69]

I recommend plugging wifi routers into a timer to help you limit screen time and frequency exposure. You may find the simple switch will help you sleep more soundly each night.

7. Reduce Stress. Lyme disease can put you into survival mode, with limited energy and debilitating symptoms to manage. Getting more efficient and intentional on how to use the energy you have will line you up for success and reduce stress.

Putting healing and self-compassion ahead of everything, and everyone else will reveal the things that are worthy of your energy. One of the first things I do with clients is to work with them on creating a daily and weekly schedule that prioritizes keeping the mind, body and home healthy, clean and nourished.

I encourage all my clients to block off an entire day each week to celebrate and acknowledge all the work put in during the week. One day off from responsibilities each week to check in with the body, listen to intuition, rest, and recharge.

Organize your medications with weekly pill organizers. Make it as easy as possible to take your medications on time. I use a combination of google calendars, phone alarm, and an erasable checklist to keep my functional hours as productive and stress-free as possible.

Try to reduce stress and self-judgment. There may be days where you seemingly accomplish very little. Never forget that every action, no matter how small, matters!

Do the best you can in each present moment and be patient with yourself. Each little step you take adds up and even if you can't see it at the time, healing is happening.

SUPPORTING DETOXIFICATION

Many Lyme patients are caught off-guard when their medications seem to make them feel worse! This happens because as some medications kill pathogens during Lyme treatment, a massive amount of toxins are released that overwhelm the body and cause an increase in symptoms. This is known as a *Jarisch-Herxheimer* reaction, more commonly referred to as a *Herx*.

A Herx reaction can not only be uncomfortable, in extreme cases it can cause seizures, strokes and heart attacks. So, it's crucial to support the body's detoxification process and monitor your symptoms throughout Lyme treatment.[70]

Of course, you don't need to be having a Herx reaction to benefit from detoxification support. Recent studies have shown that *B. burgdorferi* may consistently excrete toxins simply to ward off other bacteria, and alter its environment.[71]

As I mentioned in the How Lyme Works section, *B. burgdorferi* may also alter its environment through gene expression. Many Lyme patients who undergo genetic testing find that they have a mutation, known as MTHFR, in common.

The MTHFR gene mutation inhibits the body from processing amino acids and vitamins properly, which in turn affects the body's ability to detox.

Whether those with chronic Lyme disease had these genetic variants from birth, or if these mutations were caused by the infection is unknown.

On top of all the toxins involved in Lyme disease, our modern society is saturated with pollutants, endocrine-disrupting chemicals, processed foods, and preservatives in our everyday life.

Exposure to these daily contaminates can lead to many seemingly unconnected symptoms such as brain fog, fatigue, digestive issues, allergic reactions, trouble sleeping, skin problems, joint pain, depression, anxiety, and more.

Detoxification is the body's natural process to eliminate toxins from the body.

The human body was made to process naturally occurring toxins, largely through the skin, lungs, lymph system and liver. However, when the body is overworked from fighting Lyme disease and trying to filter the man-made toxins and irritants, supporting the body's natural process of detoxification can make a world of difference!

I know first-hand through my healing journey and work with other Lyme patients that detoxification support is crucial to help Lyme patients feel their best.

For those new to detoxification practices I've created a free guide with tips that I wish I had known from the start!

Visit my website to download a free digital copy of The Lyme Ease Herx Guidebook: A guide to help Lyme patients manage treatment reactions and symptoms today!

ww.jennhyla.com/herx-guide

Recognizing a Herx

If your symptoms worsen, or new symptoms appear within 48-hours of starting antibiotic therapy, you're likely experiencing a Herx.[72]

I remember when I would start to feel terrible within only 2 to 4 hours after treatments!

Most Lyme patients report flu-like symptoms, including headaches, swollen glands, musculoskeletal pain, fatigue, neuropathy, and brain fog. Symptoms can also include depression, anxiety, mood swings, nausea, shortness of breath, heart palpitations, and many more.

During a Herx reaction, it can be nearly impossible to think straight. Anxious thoughts begin to bubble up, and if you're anything like me, you may find yourself straight-up freaking out!

This is why it's good to have a plan in place beforehand.

Avoiding a Herx

Wouldn't it be nice to skip the whole increase in symptoms bit, and just start feeling better? While I can't promise that, I can say from personal experience and my work with other Lyme patients, that supporting the detoxification system *daily* is the best way to minimize the severity and frequency of herx reactions.

The most powerful way to support the detoxification system is by drinking plenty of high-quality filtered water throughout the day. I'm betting you've heard to drink at least 8 glasses of water per day, but did you know it also matters how you drink it?

Most of us wait until we feel pretty thirsty before taking a drink. This pang of thirst is a sign the body is already dehydrated.

When a dehydrated body gets slammed with big gulps of water, it can't process the fluid quickly enough, so it flushes right through the digestive system, and you'll likely find yourself running to the bathroom in no time. This way of drinking leaves your cells thirsty.[73]

Lyme expert, Dr. Lee Cowden recommends his patients drink 2 oz of filtered water every 15 minutes while awake to flush the cells of the body. It was a very difficult practice for me to get used to. I had to pee every fifteen minutes as my body adjusted during the first few weeks, but it was well worth the effort.

The simple act of intentionally drinking every 15 minutes improved my overall health more than anything!

Every cell in the body requires water, so support them in flushing toxins with small sips of water throughout the day. Proper hydration requires more than just fluids. Keeping a balance of electrolytes in the body is also crucial. Electrolytes are made up of sodium, potassium, calcium, bicarbonate, magnesium, chloride, phosphate.

Everyone's needs vary greatly depending on nutritional intake. Some experimentation may be needed to find the right dosage.[74]

Lymph Care

Another great way to support the detoxification process daily is through lymph massage and dry brushing. The lymphatic system is a major player in your body's immune system.

The lymph system is a network of organs and cells that work together to rid the body of waste and toxins.

It also transports fluids that contain infection-fighting white cells.[75] Modern medicine is still learning how the lymph system functions, but evidence suggests that stimulating the circulatory system and lymph system aids the body's detoxification process.[76]

A few of the ways I support my lymph system is with daily walks, yoga, lymph massage, and dry brushing. Taking a long Epsom salt bath after a few minutes of dry brushing is one of my favorite detoxification methods. It's very relaxing, reduces pain, and helps me to get a great night's sleep. I recommend adding a few essential oils and soaking for 20 minutes or more at least twice a week.

How to do a Lymph Massage

The word "massage" makes it sound more intense than it really is. The lymphatic system lies just beneath the skin, so only light pressure is required for drainage.

1. Start with 3 fingers pressing gently into the soft tissue above the collar bone close to the neck. Use a gentle pumping motion pressing in and releasing pressure for 50 repetitions. Repeat on the other side.

2. Next use flat palms and fingertips to drain the sides of the neck, beneath the ears. Gently pull the skin in downward motions parallel to the jawline for 50 repetitions.

3. Bring fingertips to the back of the neck, where the base of the skull and spine meet. Massage in a downward motion 50 times.

4. Next bring flat palms to the side of the face, placing two fingers in front of the ear, and two fingers behind. Pull gently downward 50 times.

5. Then repeat back of the neck, side of the neck, and collarbones.

How to Dry-Brush

1. Using a good-quality dry body brush, start at your feet and move upward toward your torso. You want your strokes to be long, with medium pressure so you don't hurt your skin.

2. Be sure to brush both the front and back of your legs and bottom with long, upward strokes. Brush your stomach in a circular, clockwise motion.

3. For the top half of your body, start at your hands. Move across toward the heart. Finish with your neck and chest brushing downward still toward the heart.

4. Once you are finished dry brushing, I highly recommend taking a shower to remove the dead skin cells from your body.

Managing a Herx

If you find yourself feeling worse there are many ways to support the body and ease the symptoms of a Herx reaction. I highly recommend experimenting and finding what works for you.

Once you find a few you like, write a list and keep it near your medications. It may seem silly but in the thick of a symptom storm, you might forget what works.

I find just doing one or two of these, combined with a nap does the trick for me.

1. **Take a Binder** - Activated charcoal or diatomaceous earth with lots of water. Binders help with reducing the body's inflammatory responses to toxins.

2. **Detox Tea** - A simple glass of warm water and lemon juice is great for detoxing, but you can also experiment with combining ginger, turmeric, cardamom, cinnamon, black pepper, honey or

stevia to make a comforting detox tea. You can also replace warm water with coconut milk.

3. **Detox Bath** - This is a great way to not only detox but to relax and find some relief for aches and pains. Here's my recipe for an effective detox bath:

- 4 cups Epsom salt
- 2 cups baking soda
- 1 cup apple cider vinegar
- 1 cup hydrogen peroxide
- 3 drops each of ginger, lemon, juniper berry, geranium essential oils.

Add dry ingredients and essential oils together, then slowly add all ingredients into a warm bath. Soak for 20 minutes or more. (Ginger and lemon essential oils are incredible for provoking the detoxification process, so you may find yourself sweating more than usual!)

4. **Salt Flush** - drinking around 2 tsp of salt in room temperature water as quickly as possible. This should be done on an empty stomach, and plan to stay near a bathroom for a few hours afterwards. The saltwater along with some simple yogic stretches, like knee to chest, have shown to flush the colon and digestive system. Epsom salt containers often have instructions, but any high-quality non-iodized salt can also be used.
There are contraindications, such as high blood pressure, heart problems, kidney problems, seizures, and diabetes.7 May cause stomach cramping and nausea.[77]

5. **Coffee Enema** - Enema kits are easily available online and at most pharmacies. I recommend Wilson's Organic Gold Coffee made for enemas. It lifts my brain fog, increases energy levels, eases pain, and has greatly improved my digestion.

6. **Essential Oils** - I'm a huge proponent of essential oils and their healing benefits. I add one drop of citrus essential oil to water or tea or massage it into my abdomen area. Check out my blog for a complete list of essential oils for detoxification support!

7. **Castor Oil Pack**- Be careful, it stains! Soak a thick cotton or flannel cloth in castor oil and two drops of lemon or other detoxifying essential oil (optional).

   Apply to the liver area and wrapped with plastic wrap and an elastic bandage. Castor oil works best when used with a heating pad or hot water bottle. Leave on for 20 to 60 minutes and relax during treatment.

8. **Milk Thistle** - You can take milk thistle in supplement or tea form. It has been used in traditional medicine for centuries to support and flush the liver. You should follow your intake of milk thistle with plenty of water.

9. **NAC (N-Acetyl Cysteine) Supplement** - Cysteine is the precursor amino-acid that provokes your body in creating glutathione. Glutathione is an antioxidant that facilitates the detoxification process, provides important antioxidant properties, reduces oxidative stress, and has remarkable benefits for the body.

   There are other ways to stimulate the production of glutathione. Eating a diet rich in cruciferous vegetables and supplementing with the precursor NAC may aid detoxification and reduce herxheimer reactions.[78]

10. **Breathwork** - Deep breathing exercises will calm the mind, increase oxygen to the cells, and also massage the digestive organs. I recommend lying flat on the back with one hand on the belly one hand on the chest. Breathing in and out of the mouth, fill the belly for a slow count of five. Continue breathing in to fill the chest for the count of five, and exhale

strong and long through the nose for a count of 10. Repeat this pattern for 5 to 20 minutes.

For video demonstrations of these practices download a free digital copy of *The Lyme Ease Herx Guidebook: A complete guide to help Lyme patients get through treatment reactions and symptoms*, and find more free Lyme resources on my website:

www.jennhyla.com/herx-guide

HEALING THE GUT

Gastrointestinal symptoms are common in Lyme patients, and can really inhibit healing. The latest studies are revealing fascinating links between gut health, immune health, and mental health.

Our intestines are a network of neurons, lymph nodes, and a mix of beneficial and harmful bacteria, known as the microbiome.[79]

Antibiotics and natural antimicrobials used in Lyme treatment are like swallowing a nuclear bomb to our microbiome. It wipes out all bacteria, and the effects can be seen for over 6 months after the medication is stopped.[80]

Studies indicate that balancing the microbiome with a proper diet may help to feed and replenish the immune system.[81] Eating a whole-food, anti-inflammatory diet is an important step in rebuilding the microbiome and aid in healing the gut, but there are a few more things we can do to support the healing process.

Improve digestion

To make it as easy as possible for your body to digest food, be sure to eat nutritious foods when digestive juices are highest, in the middle of the day, and always chew your food thoroughly.

Chewing not only breaks down our food, but it also stimulates the production of enzymes in our saliva that are needed to extract nutrients.[82]

When we don't chew enough it is very difficult for the body to absorb those nutrients. Studies indicate a wide variety of benefits by simply eating and chewing meals more slowly.[83]

Make it a point to intentionally chew each bite into a fine pulp before swallowing, and take a full belly breath in between bites to stimulate the digestive organs. Using digestive enzymes, like ox bile and bromelain, seem to help some patients but should be used sparingly as the body can develop a dependence on them.[84]

Consuming herb-based digestifs after meals has been recommended for centuries to support digestion. Ayurvedic medicine has recommended tea and herbal chews with ginger, cardamom, fennel, cinnamon, and cumin to aid digestion. I love enjoying a glass of ginger tea after a meal. It settles my stomach, and tastes delicious!

Address Parasites

While unpleasant to think about, parasites are living among us. According to the CDC, roughly 5%, or 16 million, Americans have been exposed to the Toxocara parasite, with millions likely going undiagnosed.[85] Toxocara and many other microscopic parasites thrive on raw food, in water, and throughout the environment.

Humans contract parasites by ingesting contaminated raw foods, inhaling airborne eggs, absorbing them through the skin, and possibly through tick bites.[86] Worldwide, and largely in low-income and rural areas, around one-sixth of the world's population are dealing with parasitic infections.[87]

Parasites can harbor tons of viruses and bacteria, muck up digestion, cause malnutrition, and inhibit healing. People with compromised immune systems are more susceptible to parasitic infections.[88]

Board-certified pathologist, and researcher, Alan B. MacDonald MD, conducted a small study where he found *B. burgdorferi*, thriving inside parasitic nematode worms, worm eggs or larvae in tissues of nineteen deceased patients.

"These microscopic worms are endosymbionts, meaning the Borrelia bacteria dwell inside the worms. A tick bite delivers the nematode into the human body."

-Alan B. MacDonald[89]

Many Lyme patients, myself included, report improvement with herbal parasite treatments and cleanses.

Address Candida & Dysbiosis

Candida is a natural yeast found in the digestive tract, mouth, and vagina. A small amount is always present and causes no symptoms in healthy individuals. Its growth is usually kept in check by the presence of the bacteria of the microbiome, and the immune system.[90]

Candida overgrowth is a common problem for Lyme patients. The antibiotics and antimicrobials commonly used for Lyme treatment are useless against this opportunistic fungus. Candida takes advantage of the space created as microbes in the gut die off and can grow out of control.[91]

Candida overgrowth can cause a long list of symptoms including brain fog, fatigue, thrush, and more. Antifungals can help keep candida in check, but this fungus feeds off sugar, so it can be extremely challenging to conquer without a completely sugar-free diet.[92]

Dysbiosis is the clinical term for an imbalance of bacteria and fungus in the gut.

A long term imbalance of these beneficial and harmful bacteria and fungi may lead to many health problems and contribute to immune deficiency.[93] It also causes inflammation of the delicate intestinal lining that often leads to increased intestinal permeability and a condition known as leaky gut. Patients with leaky gut often find themselves with a long list of symptoms, food sensitivities and severe reactions.[94]

Gut-Healing Supplements

Lyme disease did a lot of damage to my gut. I developed Small Intestinal Bacterial Overgrowth (SIBO), candida overgrowth, and leaky gut before I even began Lyme treatment. Believe me when I say I have tried countless things to heal and support my digestive system.

I wanted to include a few supplements that I believe brought me big improvements. This is not intended to be taken as medical advice.

Make sure to research, and speak to a medical professional before adding anything to your treatment protocol as some of these may have contraindications, or interact with other medications.

Here is a list of my favorite supplements for healthy gut

support:

1. **Colostrum** - Rich in immunoglobulins, which play a critical role in the healing of leaky gut syndrome. Colostrum has shown to repair damaged tissue and seal the mucus layer of the intestines.[95]

2. **Collagen** - Often referred to as the 'glue that holds us together.' Collagen is a crucial building block found in organs, muscles, skin, hair, nails, teeth, bones, blood vessels, tendons, joints, cartilage, and your digestive system. Our intestinal walls are lined with microscopic folds known as "villi" which are made of collagen. Supplementing collagen can seal leaky gut by supporting the villi's tissue growth.[96]

3. **Zinc** - An essential trace element crucial in tissue regeneration, and immune system response. Zinc deficiency is common in patients with inflammatory bowel disease and leaky gut syndrome, and has been linked to mucosal inflammation.[97]

4. **L-Glutamine** - An essential amino acid that promotes regrowth and repair to the intestinal lining. Animal studies have shown that glutamine may protect the gut from atrophy and injury under a variety of stress conditions.[98]

5. **Berberine** - This herbal supplement has been recommended for digestive issues for centuries. Animal studies show a significant reduction in inflammation and improvements in the tight junctions of the intestinal lining with berberine supplementation.[99]

6. **Marshmallow root** - This herb is widely used to ease inflammation in the stomach and digestive tract. It contains a high mucilage content which can relieve both diarrhea and constipation by creating a protective lining on the digestive tract.[100]

energy by meeting your mistakes with endless compassion. Trust that you are doing the best you can in any given moment, and cut yourself a little slack. If you wouldn't say it to your best friend, then stop saying it to yourself.

Take a look around at the world's most successful people for motivation, the majority of them have a committed mindset and visualization practice that they do daily because they know the power of the subconscious mind.

Set aside time daily to daydream and imagine what you want your life to look like when you are healed. Really allow yourself to feel and linger in the relief and joy you will feel when you reach your goals. Commit yourself to get there no matter what stands in your way.

All you need to focus on is the very next best step, and remember the words you say and think are powerful!

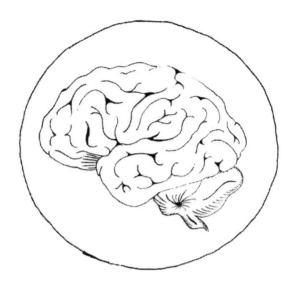

PART 3 ~ NEVER GIVE UP

Over the years I have received messages from so many people who are ready to throw in the towel and give up. I know where they are coming from.

I had a great view of rock bottom for much of my healing journey. There were many times that I wanted to give up. I literally wiped all my medications and protocols into the trash bin more than once! These moments, while terribly lonely and bleak, gave me a slap in the face to take inventory on what was working, and what needed to go.

Healing is rarely neat nor easy, you've got to be in it for the long game. Hold onto your goals and the vision of what you want your life to look like when this is all over. Start injecting confidence into each step you take.

Focus on the very next best step, and trust that it is getting you one step closer to healing.

There will likely be setbacks, mistakes, and flares. Do not let these fog your vision of the future. Lean into your intuition, and trust in your innate resilience.

Cultivate and work to strengthen the belief that you are someone who can heal from Lyme disease. That in fact, you are healing from it right now.

Each breath is an opportunity to send healing oxygen to every single cell in the body. Every bite of food is an opportunity to nourish your cells and strengthen your immune system. Every cell in the body is regenerating even as you read this.

STAY FOCUSED

One of the biggest mistakes I made along this journey was getting distracted and focusing too much energy on treating syndromes and symptoms instead of staying focused on healing from Lyme.

After I received a positive Lyme test, doctors still wanted to scan, test, poke, and prod at me even though Lyme disease could explain all of my symptoms.

I allowed myself to be referred from one specialist to another for over a year. Looking back, I think the only thing I was searching for was a doctor to say there's no permanent damage, you're going to heal from this thing! What I got instead was 15 new diagnoses, each of which were syndromes with acronyms and no known cause.

There are many ways to create a daily gratitude practice, so create one that resonates with you.

A few of my favorite gratitude practices are:

Gratitude rant: set a timer for 5 minutes, and start listing all the things you're grateful for. Either speak them out loud or write them down in a journal. Don't stop until the timer goes off!

Gratitude jar: Each time you notice something that brings a sense of appreciation or gratitude right it down and put it in a gratitude jar. At the end of the year, once a month, or just when you're feeling down read through the notes!

Stay mindful and aware of your abundance: Keep focusing your thoughts and energy towards the things that bring deep appreciation, gratitude, and self-compassion. Give yourself the time and patience to take a few full deep breaths and stay aware of each present moment. Set aside time each day to notice and acknowledge how much abundance surrounds you. No matter our hardships, there is always plenty of air to breathe, water to drink, and beauty to appreciate.

Stay inspired with Lyme patient's success stories. Many professional athletes, actors, and celebrities have publicly shared their stories in books, articles, and interviews. While reading their stories is a great pick me up, you can also find a well of inspiration and courage by looking back on all the hardships you've personally made it through.

When I take a little time, I realize that each challenging experience felt like the world was crashing down around me. Yet every single time, things eventually worked out in my favor. In fact, more often than not, I ended up more resilient because of it... so why should this time be any different?

PRIORITIZE SELF-CARE

We all have basic self-care needs such as sleeping, eating, drinking, and personal hygiene. When your energy and mobility are limited by Lyme disease, even the most basic self-care, like showering can be a challenge.

Lyme disease treatment can also come with long lists of self-care obligations. There are medications to take, appointments to make, regimens, and exercises to keep track of, all of which may leave you feeling very burnt out.

It is difficult for a healthy person to imagine how depleting these seemingly simple tasks can feel. Society's version of self-care usually involves manicures, hair salons, spas, and activities that are completely out of reach for those with chronic illness.

The kicker is when we're battling Lyme disease, feeling overwhelmed or depleted we need self-care the most!

So, below are a few of my favorite ways to practice self-care for those times when you're in pain, sick, exhausted, and stuck in bed.

Steps to create a self-care schedule:

1. Determine your non-negotiables. Create a list of your most basic self-care needs, the things you know you need to do to feel functional. For me, that means getting 8 hours of rest, taking my vitamins, eating a nutritious meal, taking a cold shower, 30-minutes of meditation, and getting dressed to shoes daily. Even if I have to crawl right back into bed afterwards, I feel best with a clean pair of clothes on. Make a list of your non-negotiables, and don't feel bad if that's all you get done for the day!

2. Develop a routine. Creating a daily routine will help you put your self-care on autopilot. Studies show it takes 66 days to form a habit, so write out your ideal routine and try to stick to it for 2 months straight![113] Building a daily routine may sound tedious, but it will help make your non-negotiables, and practicing self-care easier and ultimately free up some of your mental energy. Start by deciding what time you want to wake up and go to bed each day, then fill in your non-negotiables, appointments, and goals.

3. Master the mundane. Living with Lyme can feel like you're living in the movie Groundhog's Day, completing the same mundane tasks day in and day out. With limited energy, you may find yourself feeling resentful towards your daily tasks.

See if you can invite curiosity and a little fun into your day. I like to set a timer and see how quickly I can organize my medications, or put my laundry away each week. I also enjoy listening to a motivational podcast, or audiobook while completing chores. Find little ways to make your mundane tasks feel more exciting!

4. Create a list of self-care go-to's. When you're feeling overwhelmed the last thing you need is to try and read through a bunch of blogs on self-care!

Have a list or a box of things that bring you emotional and physical comfort ready before those hard days come around! This can include your favorite movie, songs, snacks, essential oils, or anything really!

Below are a few of my favorite self-care go-to's.

1. Hydrate! Dehydration can cause heaps of seemingly unrelated symptoms! Clinical studies have shown that many people interpret feelings of thirst as hunger![114] Meaning we are reaching for snacks when we ought to reach for a glass of water. Most of us wait until we are already dehydrated to take a drink. Next time you're feeling overwhelmed, try reaching for a big glass of water.

2. Breathwork. Taking short shallow breaths throughout the day can cause headaches, irritability, digestive issues, neck and shoulder tension, and a long list of seemingly unrelated symptoms. When I'm feeling overwhelmed a few minutes of breathwork can shift everything!

One simple practice is to breathe in through the nose for the count of 4, retain the breath for the count of 7, and exhale strongly through the nose for a count of 8. Repeat this breathing pattern for 5 to 10 minutes for relaxing effects.

3. Gentle Movement. The body was made for movement! Staying stagnant for long periods of time can impact the physical and emotional body. Gentle movement every few hours will increase blood flow, oxygen, and energy! Just a few minutes of gentle stretching can move stagnant energy, and give the day a new perspective. Try some simple yoga postures like reclined twist, and cat-cow, that can be done in bed to get your body moving.

4. Journaling. With the stress of chronic illness, and our eyes glued to social media, it's easy to feel overwhelmed. Taking a few

Be aware that there is a lot of misinformation circulating about Lyme disease. Make sure you check references and even cross-reference information.

I recommend using the search engine scholar.google.com to search through peer-reviewed scientific studies from around the world.

Even if you don't understand the science you can get a good idea of what was done, and what they found by reading the summary section, and the conclusion. Make sure to check for bias by reading the conflict of interest and funding statements also.

When I was first reading up on Lyme disease, I read nothing else! I completely immersed myself in Facebook groups, blogs, and online seminars. I highly recommend **not** doing that while trying to heal.

Stay focused on healing, get support, take breaks, and research from peer-reviewed scientific sources.

I hope that the information in this book will be helpful along your healing journey.

Remember that anytime you have setbacks or flares you can come back to this information.

Visit my website for a free Lyme 101 video class, free Herx guidebook, and more resources to help you kick Lyme disease's butt!

www.jennhyla.com/resources

You will find more reputable resources on Lyme disease on the next few pages for your convenience.

Lyme Education Websites

- International Lyme and Associated Disease Society
https://www.ilads.org/research-literature/

- Global Lyme Alliance https://globallymealliance.org/

- Lyme Disease Association:
https://lymediseaseassociation.org/

- Bay Area Lyme Foundation:
https://www.bayarealyme.org/about-lyme/

- Lyme Knowledge http://www.lymeknowledge.com/

Lyme Education Books

- *Healing Lyme, Natural Healing and Prevention of Lyme Borreliosis and Its Coinfections* by Dr. Stephen Buhner

- *How can I get better? An Action Plan for Treating Resistant Lyme & Chronic Disease* by Dr. Richard Horowitz

- *New Paradigms in Lyme Disease Treatment. 10 Top Doctors Reveal Strategies That Work* by Connie Strasheim

- *Bitten. The Secret History of Lyme Disease and Biological Weapons* by Kris Newby

9. Buhner, Stephen. (2005). Healing Lyme: natural prevention and treatment of Lyme borreliosis and its coinfections. Randolph, VT: Raven Press. (pp 25)

10. Buhner, Stephen (2005). Healing Lyme: natural prevention and treatment of Lyme borreliosis and its coinfections. Randolph, VT: Raven Press. (pp 24)

11. Wang, Guiqing. 2015. Chapter 104 *Borrelia burgdorferi* and Other Borrelia Species. Molecular Medical Microbiology.Elsevier Ltd.

12. TickEncounter Resource Center. (n.d.). Retrieved from https://tickencounter.org/tick_identification/tick_species

13. Middelveen, M. J., Burke, J., Sapi, E., Bandoski, C., Filush, K. R., Wang, Y., et al. (2014, December 18). Culture and identification of Borrelia spirochetes in human vaginal and seminal secretions. Retrieved from https://www.ncbi.nlm.nih.gov/pubmed/28713539

14. Rudenko, N., Golovchenko, M., Kybicova, K. et al. (2019). Metamorphoses of Lyme disease spirochetes: phenomenon of Borrelia persisters. Parasites Vectors 12, 237. Retrieved from https://doi.org/10.1186/s13071-019-3495-7

15. Bernard, Q., Smith, A. A., Yang, X., et al. (2018, April 17). Plasticity in early immune evasion strategies of a bacterial pathogen. Retrieved from https://www.pnas.org/content/115/16/E3788#abstract-2

16. Bernard, Quentin, Smith, Alexis A., Yang, Xiuli, et al. (2018, April). Plasticity in early immune evasion strategies of a bacterial pathogen. Proceedings of the National Academy of Sciences 115 (16) E3788-E3797. Retrieved from https://www.pnas.org/content/115/16/E3788#abstract-2

17. Meriläinen, L., Herranen, A., Schwarzbach, A., & Gilbert, L. (2015). Morphological and biochemical features of *Borrelia burgdorferi* pleomorphic forms. Microbiology (Reading, England), 161(Pt 3), 516–527. https://doi.org/10.1099/mic.0.000027

18. Di Domenico, E. G., Cavallo, I., Bordignon, V., D'Agosto, G., Pontone, M., Trento, E., Gallo, M. T., Prignano, G., Pimpinelli, F., Toma, L., & Ensoli, F. (2018). The Emerging Role of Microbial Biofilm in Lyme Neuroborreliosis. Frontiers in neurology, 9, 1048. https://doi.org/10.3389/fneur.2018.01048

19. Sapi,E., Balasubramanian, K, Poruri, A, et al. (2016). Evidence Of In Vivo Existence Of Borrelia Biofilm In Borrelial Lymphocytomas. European Journal of Microbiology and Immunology 6, P 9–24. Retrieved from https://akademiai.com/doi/pdf/10.1556/1886.2015.00049

20. Rudenko, N., Golovchenko, M., Kybicova, K. et al. (2019). Metamorphoses of Lyme disease spirochetes: phenomenon of Borrelia persisters. Parasites Vectors 12, 237. Retrieved from https://doi.org/10.1186/s13071-019-3495-7

21. Miller, Bob CTN (2016). Higher Levels of Genetic Variants (SNPs) Found in those with Chronic Lyme Disease. NutriGenetic Research Institute. Retrieved from https://static1.squarespace.com/static/5cc1b2259d4149175b931ed4/t/5cc21eda15fcc03c556aa9b5/1556225755536/NGRI_Chronic-LymeDNA-ResearchStudy.pdf

22. Lyme Disease Testing. (n.d.). Retrieved from https://globallymealliance.org/about-lyme/diagnosis/testing/

23. Mead P, Petersen J, Hinckley A. (2019, August 15). Updated CDC Recommendation for Serologic Diagnosis of Lyme Disease. MMWR Morb Mortal Wkly Rep 2019;68:703. Retrieved from https://www.cdc.gov/mmwr/volumes/68/wr/mm6832a4.htm?s_cid=mm6832a4_

24. About Lyme. (n.d.). Retrieved from https://globallymealliance.org/about-lyme/

25. Diagnosis and Testing. (2019, November 20). Retrieved from https://www.cdc.gov/lyme/diagnosistesting/index.html

26. Aguero-Rosenfeld, M. E., Wang, G., Schwartz, I., & Wormser, G. P. (2005, July). Diagnosis of lyme borreliosis. Retrieved from https://www.ncbi.nlm.nih.gov/pmc/articles/PMC1195970/

27. Laboratory tests that are not recommended. (2018, December 21). Retrieved from https://www.cdc.gov/lyme/diagnosistesting/labtest/otherlab/index.ht ml

28. People with Lyme disease co-infections experience more severe illness. (n.d.). Retrieved from https://www.lymedisease.org/lyme-basics/co-infections/about-co-infections/

29. Lyme Disease: Introduction to Symptoms, Diagnosis and Treatment. (n.d.). Retrieved from https://www.lymedisease.org/lyme-basics/lyme-disease/about-lyme/

30. Wormser, P., G., Dattwyler, et al. (2006, November 1). Clinical Assessment, Treatment, and Prevention of Lyme Disease, Human Granulocytic Anaplasmosis, and Babesiosis: Clinical Practice Guidelines by the Infectious Diseases Society of America. Retrieved from https://academic.oup.com/cid/article/43/9/1089/422463#74156512

31. Post-Treatment Lyme Disease Syndrome. (2019, November 8). Retrieved from https://www.cdc.gov/lyme/postlds/index.html

32. Webster, L., & Donna. (2018, June 8). Why Is Chronic Lyme Disease Controversial? Retrieved from http://www.lynnwebstermd.com/chronic-lyme-disease-controversial/

33. Everything about Lyme disease is steeped in controversy. Now some doctors are too afraid to treat patients. (2019, October 1). Retrieved from https://www.ilads.org/everything-about-lyme-disease-is-steeped-in-controversy-now-some-doctors-are-too-afraid-to-treat-patients/

34. New Scan Technique Reveals Brain Inflammation Associated with Post-Treatment Lyme disease Syndrome. (2019, February 5). Retrieved from https://www.hopkinsmedicine.org/news/newsroom/news-releases/new-scan-technique-reveals-brain-inflammation-associated-with-post-treatment-lyme-disease-syndrome

35. Research & Literature. (n.d.). Retrieved from https://www.ilads.org/research-literature/

36. Fallon, B. A., & Nields, J. A. (1994, November). Lyme disease: a neuropsychiatric illness. Retrieved from https://www.ncbi.nlm.nih.gov/pubmed/7943444

Part 2 – Lyme Treatment Options

37. Rudenko, N., Golovchenko, M., Kybicova, K. et al. (2019). Metamorphoses of Lyme disease spirochetes: phenomenon of Borrelia persisters. Parasites Vectors 12, 237. Retrieved from https://doi.org/10.1186/s13071-019-3495-7

38. Maloy, A. L., Black, R. D., & Segurola, R. J. (1998). Lyme disease complicated by the Jarisch-Herxheimer reaction. Retrieved from https://www.ncbi.nlm.nih.gov/pubmed/9610974

39. Lyme Disease Co-Infection. (n.d.). Retrieved from https://www.niaid.nih.gov/diseases-conditions/lyme-disease-co-infection

40. ILADS Treatment Guidelines. (n.d.). Retrieved from https://www.ilads.org/patient-care/ilads-treatment-guidelines/

41. Horowitz, R. (2017). How Can I Get Better? An Action Plan for Treating Resistant Lyme & Chronic Disease. St Martin's Press. New York, NY (pp 69 -81)

42. Hub. Staff. (2018, December 4). Essential oils from garlic, herbs kill persistent Lyme disease bacteria. Retrieved from https://hub.jhu.edu/2018/12/04/lyme-disease-treatment-essential-oils/

43. Human Herpesvirus 6: An Emerging Pathogen - Volume 5, Number 3-June 1999 - Emerging Infectious Diseases journal - CDC. (n.d.). Retrieved from https://wwwnc.cdc.gov/eid/article/5/3/99-0306_article

44. Craig Freudenrich, Ph.D. (2019, Oct 10). "How Viruses Work" Retrieved from https://science.howstuffworks.com/life/cellular-microscopic/virus-human.htm

45. Stiller, M., Pak, G. H., Shupack, J., Thaler, S., Kenny, C., & Jondreau, L. (2006, July 29). A portable pulsed electromagnetic field (PEMF) device to enhance healing of recalcitrant venous ulcers: a double-blind, placebo-controlled clinical trial. Retrieved from https://onlinelibrary.wiley.com/doi/abs/10.1111/j.1365-2133.1992.tb08047.x

46. Acupuncture: In Depth. (2017, February 21). Retrieved from https://nccih.nih.gov/health/acupuncture/introduction

47. Miana, V. V., & González, E. A. P. (2018, March 28). Adipose tissue stem cells in regenerative medicine. Retrieved from https://www.ncbi.nlm.nih.gov/pmc/articles/PMC5880231/

48. Trafton, A., & MIT News Office. (2018, May 3). Fasting boosts stem cells' regenerative capacity. Retrieved from http://news.mit.edu/2018/fasting-boosts-stem-cells-regenerative-capacity-0503

49. FoundMyFitness Topic - Fasting. (n.d.). Retrieved from https://www.foundmyfitness.com/topics/fasting#transformative-effects-of-fasting

50. Cunningham, A. B., Lennox, J. E., & Ross, R. J. (2010). A Brief History of Biofilms. Retrieved from

https://www.cs.montana.edu/webworks/projects/stevesbook/contents
/chapters/chapter001/section003/blue/page001.html

51. Donlan, R. M. (2002, September). Biofilms: microbial life on
    surfaces. Retrieved from
    https://www.ncbi.nlm.nih.gov/pmc/articles/PMC2732559/

52. Stewart, P. S. (2002, July). Mechanisms of antibiotic resistance in
    bacterial biofilms. Retrieved from
    https://www.ncbi.nlm.nih.gov/pubmed/12195733

53. Lacout, A., Dacher, V., El Hajjam, M., Marcy, P. Y., & Perronne, C.
    (2018, March). Biofilms busters to improve the detection of Borrelia
    using PCR. Retrieved from
    https://www.ncbi.nlm.nih.gov/pubmed/29447935

54. Okin, D., & Medzhitov, R. (2012, September 10). Evolution of
    Inflammatory Diseases. Retrieved from
    https://www.sciencedirect.com/science/article/pii/S09609822120082
    02

55. Kiecolt-Glaser, J. K. (2010, May). Stress, food, and inflammation:
    psychoneuroimmunology and nutrition at the cutting edge. Retrieved
    from https://www.ncbi.nlm.nih.gov/pmc/articles/PMC2868080/

56. Baltimore. (n.d.). University of Maryland Graduate School.
    Retrieved from https://graduate.umaryland.edu/gsa/gazette/February-
    2016/How-the-human-body-uses-electricity/

57. Chevalier, G., Sinatra, S. T., Oschman, J. L., Sokal, K., & Sokal, P.
    (2012). Earthing: health implications of reconnecting the human
    body to the Earth's surface electrons. Retrieved from
    https://www.ncbi.nlm.nih.gov/pmc/articles/PMC3265077/

58. Oschman, J. L., Chevalier, G., & Brown, R. (2015, March 24). The
    effects of grounding (earthing) on inflammation, the immune
    response, wound healing, and prevention and treatment of chronic
    inflammatory and autoimmune diseases. Retrieved from
    https://www.ncbi.nlm.nih.gov/pmc/articles/PMC4378297/

59. Neuroscience News. (2019, April 4). 20 Minute Contact with Nature Reduces Stress Hormone Cortisol. Retrieved from https://neurosciencenews.com/nature-cortisol-stress-11001/?fbclid=IwAR1hWB67tfUTeVvuPOYMUyxWjCrBHed0n7k XIAM9823RelxPr4FoJSRy1J4

60. Mooventhan, A., & Nivethitha, L. (2014, May). Scientific evidence-based effects of hydrotherapy on various systems of the body. Retrieved from https://www.ncbi.nlm.nih.gov/pmc/articles/PMC4049052/

61. Shevchuk, N. A. (2008). Adapted cold shower as a potential treatment for depression. Retrieved from https://www.ncbi.nlm.nih.gov/pubmed/17993252

62. How eating feeds into the body clock. (2019, April 25). Retrieved from https://www.sciencedaily.com/releases/2019/04/190425143607.htm

63. FoundMyFitness Topic - Fasting. (n.d.). Retrieved from https://www.foundmyfitness.com/topics/fasting

64. Czeisler, Charles A. (2015, March) Duration, timing and quality of sleep are each vital for health, performance and safety. Sleep Health: Journal of the National Sleep Foundation, Volume 1, Issue 1, 5 – 8. Retrieved from https://www.sleephealthjournal.org/article/S2352-7218(14)00013-8/fulltext

65. Bryant, P. A., Trinder, J., & Curtis, N. (n.d.). Sick and tired: does sleep have a vital role in the immune system? Retrieved from https://www.nature.com/articles/nri1369

66. Corey, S. M., Epel, E., & et al. (2014, November). Effect of restorative yoga vs. stretching on diurnal cortisol dynamics and psychosocial outcomes in individuals with the metabolic syndrome: the PRYSMS randomized controlled trial. Retrieved from https://www.ncbi.nlm.nih.gov/pmc/articles/PMC4174464/

67. Harvard Health Publishing. (n.d.). Blue light has a dark side. Retrieved from https://www.health.harvard.edu/staying-healthy/blue-light-has-a-dark-side

68. McCarthy-Jones, S. (2019, September 2). Social networking sites may be controlling your mind – here's how to take charge. Retrieved from https://theconversation.com/social-networking-sites-may-be-controlling-your-mind-heres-how-to-take-charge-88516

69. Pall, M. L. (2018, March 21). Wi-Fi is an important threat to human health. Retrieved from https://www.sciencedirect.com/science/article/pii/S0013935118300355#!

70. Butler T. (2017). The Jarisch-Herxheimer Reaction After Antibiotic Treatment of Spirochetal Infections: A Review of Recent Cases and Our Understanding of Pathogenesis. The American journal of tropical medicine and hygiene, 96(1), 46–52. https://doi.org/10.4269/ajtmh.16-0434

71. Molloy, E.M., Casjens, S.R., Cox, C.L. et al. (2015) Identification of the minimal cytolytic unit for streptolysin S and an expansion of the toxin family. BMC Microbiol 15, 141). https://doi.org/10.1186/s12866-015-0464-y

72. Herxheimer Reaction. (n.d.). Retrieved from https://www.sciencedirect.com/topics/immunology-and-microbiology/herxheimer-reaction

73. Cozean, N., & Dpt. (2018, February 1). Sipping vs. Gulping: HOW you drink may matter more than HOW MUCH. Retrieved from https://www.pelvicsanity.com/single-post/2018/01/31/Sipping-vs-Gulping-HOW-you-drink-may-matter-more-than-HOW-MUCH

74. Felman, A. (2017, November 20). Everything you need to know about electrolytes. Retrieved from https://www.medicalnewstoday.com/articles/153188

defenses. Bacteriological reviews, 30(2), 442–459. Retrieved from
https://www.ncbi.nlm.nih.gov/pmc/articles/PMC441005/pdf/bactrev
00193-0187.pdf

92. Man, A., Ciurea, C. N., Pasaroiu, D., Savin, A.-I., et al. (2017,
September). New perspectives on the nutritional factors influencing
growth rate of Candida albicans in diabetics. An in vitro study.
Retrieved from
https://www.ncbi.nlm.nih.gov/pmc/articles/PMC5572443/

93. Peterson, C. T., Sharma, V., Elmén, L., & Peterson, S. N. (2015,
February 16). Immune homeostasis, dysbiosis and therapeutic
modulation of the gut microbiota. Retrieved from
https://onlinelibrary.wiley.com/doi/full/10.1111/cei.12474

94. Obrenovich, M. E. M. (2018, October 18). Leaky Gut, Leaky Brain?
Retrieved from
https://www.ncbi.nlm.nih.gov/pmc/articles/PMC6313445/

95. Stone, T. E. (n.d.). Colostrum Heals Leaky Gut Syndrome! Retrieved
from https://immunetreesa.co.za/files/Colostrum Heals Leaky Gut
Syndrome.pdf

96. Myers, A. (2019, November 13). The Top 7 Health Benefits of
Collagen. Retrieved from
https://www.amymyersmd.com/2019/06/the-top-7-benefits-of-
collagen/

97. Rubin, T., D., Gulotta, George, et al. (2016, December 7). Zinc
Deficiency is Associated with Poor Clinical Outcomes in Patients
with Inflammatory Bowel Disease. Retrieved from
https://academic.oup.com/ibdjournal/article/23/1/152/4595539?searc
hresult=1

98. Wang, B., Wu, G., Zhou, Z. et al. (2015). Glutamine and intestinal
barrier function. Amino Acids 47, 2143–2154. Retrieved from
https://doi.org/10.1007/s00726-014-1773-4

99. Amasheh, M., Fromm, A., Krug, S. M., Amasheh, S., et al. (2010, December 1). TNFα-induced and berberine-antagonized tight junction barrier impairment via tyrosine kinase, Akt and NFκB signaling. Retrieved from https://jcs.biologists.org/content/123/23/4145.long#sec-15

100. Myers, A. (2018, October 10). 8 Supplements To Heal A Leaky Gut. Retrieved from https://www.mindbodygreen.com/0-9336/8-supplements-to-heal-a-leaky-gut.html

101. Peterson, C. T., Sharma, V., Uchitel, S., Denniston, K., Chopra, D., et al. (2018, July). Prebiotic Potential of Herbal Medicines Used in Digestive Health and Disease. Retrieved from https://www.ncbi.nlm.nih.gov/pmc/articles/PMC6065514/

102. Ghalayani, P., Emami, H., Pakravan, F., & Isfahani, M. N. (2014, October 28). Comparison of triamcinolone acetonide mucoadhesive film with licorice mucoadhesive film on radiotherapy-induced oral mucositis: A randomized double-blinded clinical trial. Retrieved from https://onlinelibrary.wiley.com/doi/abs/10.1111/ajco.12295

103. Lamprecht, M., Bogner, S., Schippinger, G. et al. (2012) Probiotic supplementation affects markers of intestinal barrier, oxidation, and inflammation in trained men; a randomized, double-blinded, placebo-controlled trial. J Int Soc Sports Nutr 9, 45. https://doi.org/10.1186/1550-2783-9-45

104. Dispenza, J. (2015). You are the placebo: making your mind matter. Carlsbad, CA: Hay House, Inc.

105. Littrell, J. (2008). The mind-body connection: Not just a theory anymore. Social Work in Health Care, 46(4), 17-38. Retrieved from https://scholarworks.gsu.edu/cgi/viewcontent.cgi?referer=&httpsredir=1&article=1050&context=ssw_facpub

106. Harvard Health Publishing. (n.d.). The power of the placebo effect. Retrieved from https://www.health.harvard.edu/mental-health/the-power-of-the-placebo-effect

107.   News Center. (n.d.). Patient mindset matters in healing and deserves more study, experts say. Retrieved from https://med.stanford.edu/news/all-news/2017/03/health-care-providers-should-harness-power-of-mindsets.html

Part 3 – Never Give Up

108.   News Center. (n.d.). Patient mindset matters in healing and deserves more study, experts say. Retrieved from https://med.stanford.edu/news/all-news/2017/03/health-care-providers-should-harness-power-of-mindsets.html

109.   Baumeister, R. F., & Tierney, J. (2012). Willpower: rediscovering the greatest human strength. New York: Penguin Books.

110.   What you need to know about willpower: The psychological science of self-control. (n.d.). Retrieved from https://www.apa.org/helpcenter/willpower

111.   The Healing Power of Gratitude. (n.d.). Retrieved from https://www.psychologytoday.com/us/blog/compassion-matters/201511/the-healing-power-gratitude

112.   Allen, S. (2018, May). The Science of Gratitude. Retrieved from https://ggsc.berkeley.edu/images/uploads/GGSC-JTF_White_Paper-Gratitude-FINAL.pdf

113.   Lally, P., Van Jaarsveld, C., Potts, H., & Wardle, J. (2009, July 16). How are habits formed: Modelling habit formation in the real world. Retrieved from http://repositorio.ispa.pt/bitstream/10400.12/3364/1/IJSP_998-1009.pdf

114.   James, A. (2018, February 5). Hunger vs. thirst: tips to tell the difference. Retrieved from https://pkdcure.org/blog/hunger-vs-thirst/

115.   Gaia Staff. (n.d.). The Benefits of Chanting: Reclaim the Powers of Creation. Retrieved from https://www.gaia.com/article/benefits-of-chanting

ACKNOWLEDGMENTS

Over the moon, heart-bursting gratitude to my family, friends, mentors, supporters, and guides who made this book and this life possible.

A very special thank you to my soul sister, Courtney Carroll for creating the beautiful cover art and graphic design. Big, big thank you to my brother for reading through and editing the *really* rough drafts, and not even making fun of me!

Thank you to Rena, at P.ink Content Solutions, who helped me focus and polish my message with compassion, you are simply the best.

There is no adequate way to thank all the Lyme survivors, doctors, and advocates who have dedicated blood, sweat, and tears to cultivating awareness, support, and advocating for patient rights. You are all warriors.

Immense gratitude to Gregg Kirk, at the Ticked Off Foundation. Thank you for never hesitating to offer support and guidance to me, and for your wonderful review.

A heart-filled thank you to Lauren Lovejoy, at Lyme Warrior. Thank you for taking the time to review my book, your unwavering support of the Lyme community is awe inspiring. My deepest appreciation to Bre Armstrong, thank you for your unstoppable encouragement and support.

I cannot go without offering my sincere gratitude to all the scientists, doctors, and researchers, doing the dirty work to dig through the controversies and politics in hopes of uncovering a cure for this complex illness. Godspeed.

ABOUT THE AUTHOR

Jenn Hyla is a speaker, Lyme advocate and recovery coach. Her experiences as a field biologist healing from and mentoring those with Lyme provides new perspectives, science-backed alternative treatment options, and aims to help others skip the mistakes she made during her inspiring healing journey.

A yogi at heart, she believes you can find well-being at this present moment no matter what state you are in. When she's not writing and researching you will find Jenn in nature taking walks, painting, reading, practicing yoga, and petting strangers' dogs.

Printed in Great Britain
by Amazon

78647194R00066